FOOD JOURNAL

Name_____

Phone_____

Notes

Breakfast

Lunch

Dinner

Snacks

Water

Breakfast

Lunch

Dinner

Snacks

Water

_____

Breakfast

Lunch

Dinner

Snacks	Water

_____

Breakfast

Lunch

Dinner

Snacks	Water

_____

Breakfast

Lunch

Dinner

Snacks	Water

_____

Breakfast

Lunch

Dinner

Snacks	Water

_____

Breakfast

Lunch

Dinner

Snacks	Water

Breakfast

Lunch

Dinner

Snacks

Water

Breakfast

Lunch

Dinner

Snacks	Water

_____

Breakfast

Lunch

Dinner

Snacks

Water

_____

Breakfast

Lunch

Dinner

Snacks	Water

Breakfast

Lunch

Dinner

Snacks

Water

_____

Breakfast

Lunch

Dinner

Snacks	Water

_____

Breakfast

Lunch

Dinner

Snacks	Water

Breakfast

Lunch

Dinner

Snacks

Water

Breakfast

Lunch

Dinner

Snacks

Water

Breakfast

Lunch

Dinner

Snacks	Water

_____

Breakfast

Lunch

Dinner

Snacks	Water

_____

Breakfast

Lunch

Dinner

Snacks	Water

Breakfast

Lunch

Dinner

Snacks

Water

_____

Breakfast

Lunch

Dinner

Snacks

Water

Breakfast

Lunch

Dinner

Snacks

Water

_____

Breakfast

Lunch

Dinner

Snacks	Water

_____

Breakfast

Lunch

Dinner

Snacks	Water

_____

Breakfast

Lunch

Dinner

Snacks	Water

_____

Breakfast

Lunch

Dinner

Snacks	Water

_____

Breakfast

Lunch

Dinner

Snacks	Water

_____

Breakfast

Lunch

Dinner

Snacks	Water

_____

Breakfast

Lunch

Dinner

Snacks

Water

_____

Breakfast

Lunch

Dinner

Snacks	Water

Breakfast

Lunch

Dinner

Snacks

Water

_____

Breakfast

Lunch

Dinner

Snacks	Water

_____

Breakfast

Lunch

Dinner

Snacks

Water

_____

Breakfast

Lunch

Dinner

Snacks	Water

_____

Breakfast

Lunch

Dinner

Snacks	Water

_____

Breakfast

Lunch

Dinner

Snacks

Water

_____

Breakfast

Lunch

Dinner

Snacks	Water

_____

Breakfast

Lunch

Dinner

Snacks	Water

_____

Breakfast

Lunch

Dinner

Snacks	Water

_____

Breakfast

Lunch

Dinner

Snacks	Water

_____

Breakfast

Lunch

Dinner

Snacks	Water

_____

Breakfast

Lunch

Dinner

Snacks	Water

_____

Breakfast

Lunch

Dinner

Snacks	Water

_____

Breakfast

Lunch

Dinner

Snacks	Water

_____

Breakfast

Lunch

Dinner

Snacks	Water

Breakfast

Lunch

Dinner

Snacks

Water

_____

Breakfast

Lunch

Dinner

Snacks

Water

_____

Breakfast

Lunch

Dinner

Snacks	Water

_____

Breakfast

Lunch

Dinner

Snacks

Water

_____

Breakfast

Lunch

Dinner

Snacks	Water

_____

Breakfast

Lunch

Dinner

Snacks

Water

Breakfast

Lunch

Dinner

Snacks	Water

_____

Breakfast

Lunch

Dinner

Snacks	Water

_____

Breakfast

Lunch

Dinner

Snacks	Water

_____

Breakfast

Lunch

Dinner

Snacks

Water

Breakfast

Lunch

Dinner

Snacks

Water

_____

Breakfast

Lunch

Dinner

Snacks	Water

_____

Breakfast

Lunch

Dinner

Snacks	Water

_____

Breakfast

Lunch

Dinner

Snacks	Water

_____

Breakfast

Lunch

Dinner

Snacks	Water

_____

Breakfast

Lunch

Dinner

Snacks	Water

Breakfast

Lunch

Dinner

Snacks

Water

Breakfast

Lunch

Dinner

Snacks

Water

Breakfast

Lunch

Dinner

Snacks

Water

_____

Breakfast

Lunch

Dinner

Snacks	Water

_____

Breakfast

Lunch

Dinner

Snacks

Water

_____

Breakfast

Lunch

Dinner

Snacks

Water

Breakfast

Lunch

Dinner

Snacks

Water

_____

Breakfast

Lunch

Dinner

Snacks

Water

_____

Breakfast

Lunch

Dinner

Snacks	Water

_____

Breakfast

Lunch

Dinner

Snacks

Water

Breakfast

Lunch

Dinner

Snacks

Water

_____

Breakfast

Lunch

Dinner

Snacks

Water

Breakfast

Lunch

Dinner

Snacks

Water

_____

Breakfast

Lunch

Dinner

Snacks	Water

Breakfast

Lunch

Dinner

Snacks

Water

_____

Breakfast

Lunch

Dinner

Snacks	Water

Breakfast

Lunch

Dinner

Snacks

Water

_____

Breakfast

Lunch

Dinner

Snacks

Water

_____

Breakfast

Lunch

Dinner

Snacks	Water

_____

Breakfast

Lunch

Dinner

Snacks

Water

_____

Breakfast

Lunch

Dinner

Snacks

Water

_____

Breakfast

Lunch

Dinner

Snacks	Water

Breakfast

Lunch

Dinner

Snacks

Water

_____

Breakfast

Lunch

Dinner

Snacks	Water

_____

Breakfast

Lunch

Dinner

Snacks	Water

_____

Breakfast

Lunch

Dinner

Snacks	Water

Breakfast

Lunch

Dinner

Snacks

Water

_____

Breakfast

Lunch

Dinner

Snacks	Water

_____

Breakfast

Lunch

Dinner

Snacks

Water

Made in the USA
Columbia, SC
12 October 2024

44149198R00057